Alka

Drink Your Way to Vibrant Health, Massive Energy and Natural Weight Loss

By Marta Tuchowska
Copyright ©Marta Tuchowska 2015, 2019

www.HolisticWellnessProject.com

"*ALKALINE SMOOTHIES*" WILL TEACH YOU HOW TO INCORPORATE MORE ALKALINE RAW FOODS INTO YOUR DIET TO ENJOY HIGH ENERGY LEVELS, HOLISTIC WELLNESS, AND NATURAL WEIGHT LOSS.

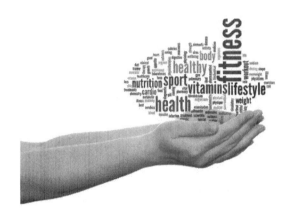

The book is not intended to provide medical advice or to take the place of medical advice and treatment from your personal physician. Readers are advised to consult their own doctors or other qualified health professionals regarding the treatment of medical conditions. The author shall not be held liable or responsible for any misunderstanding or misuse of the information contained in this book. The information is not intended to diagnose, treat or cure any disease.

Contents

Restoring Your Energy Levels

Imagine feeling like you are 18 again. Imagine a life without aches, pains, excess weight, and stiffness. Imagine feeling light, happy, and energized.

What choices have you made about your wellbeing?
Do you bounce out of bed in the mornings, or do you continue pressing the snooze button for just a few more moments of sleep? Are you able to get through the day without feeling fatigued?

Do you suffer from any ailments? Can't lose weight even though you count calories and follow the latest "dieting" fad?

Here's the good news: **you don't have to continue suffering**. But...

You have to *make a choice*. Choose to commit to doing what it takes to get healthy, have more energy, and create a body that you want. It's all about commitment and simple, healthy habits.

This is what this book is all about. Alkaline smoothies are a great, holistic tool to help you nourish your body and mind to achieve your health goals so you can be the person you want to be.

They are a great way to add more healthy, alkaline foods into your diet that will help you eradicate:

- Lack of energy
- Mental fog
- Excess Weight

It doesn't matter if you are Paleo, vegan, or gluten-free. You can always add more alkaline foods into your diet, and alkaline smoothies are the best way to do it. All the recipes from this book are *100% vegan, dairy-free, gluten-free, and soy-free.* I have included a myriad of different recipes with different ingredients to make sure I accommodate different nutritional and taste preferences.

I am pleased to present recipes that are also compatible with a Paleo Diet (Vegan-Paleo).

Perhaps you suffer from fatigue and stiffness, or perhaps you would like to lose weight. Perhaps you feel that you are simply ageing, and you need to expect to feel not-so-good anymore.

If that's the case, you have the power to change it.

Your body might be feeling sick and tired because of what you've been putting into it (processed foods, sugar, caffeine, poor quality water, stress, alcohol, yeast, bacteria, tobacco, gluten, drugs, negative emotions, too many animal products...). Add to it: pollution and not enough sleep and lack of physical activity.

It makes sense that if you attend the root cause of the problem by implementing a lifestyle rich in nutrient dense, alkaline forming foods, you will naturally take care of what plagues you.

My editor, Claire, is a 41 year old professional woman who suffered from obesity, migraines, digestive problems, rashes, low immunity and inflammation for many years. As a result of her overly acidic body from all the poor food choices she made, she experienced tremendous pain from gastric reflux, so much so that her doctor wanted to operate on her.

But once she started following an alkaline diet, she stopped having gastric reflux pain and began losing weight without feeling deprived. She also found more energy to get more done each day. She's happy with her new balanced lifestyle as she suddenly has more energy and time to spend with her children. She keeps experimenting with new alkaline recipes as she wants her family to eat in a healthy way too. She feels more productive with her work and is able to provide better services for her clients. And the best part is that she finally stopped counting calories! She loves eating and she eats 5 times a day.

People who have changed their diets to an alkaline diet experience huge benefits, and there are plenty of real-life stories to back it up. I, myself, have witnessed tremendous changes in my own health and wellbeing; the alkaline diet combined with other treatments, and lifestyle changes have helped cure my eye of uveitis (inflammation of the uvea, very often caused by autoimmune disorders) which is a serious eye disease that can even result in blindness.

I have also experienced a myriad of other benefits. This is why I am writing this book. I want to show you the practical way of enriching your diet with nutrient-packed, alkaline foods so that you can FEEL it yourself.

To be honest with you, unlike other diets I have tried, the alkaline diet totally met my demands. I felt better and better every day. Physically, mentally and emotionally. The Alkaline Diet is the best holistic beauty treatment you can get. It helps you glow. If you happen to have any skin problems, or wish to 'look healthier', the alkaline approach is the way to go.

High energy levels? You bet! I am brimming with energy. If you do the alkaline diet, your energy levels have no choice but to go up. Seriously, I am an active person and I just love getting more and more stuff done. The alkaline lifestyle was one of the best things I have done for myself and I just can't recommend it enough. All I had to do was to learn how to add more alkalizing foods into my diet and how to ban or reduce acidic foods.

I had to go through a process of creating and organizing a new way of life. This is how I managed to burn excess fat and achieve my ideal weight without feeling deprived (I am a foodie!). I also feel stronger and hardly ever get colds of flu. Even if I do, it's so mild that I don't feel affected at all and it goes away quickly.

Here is the truth: we can't expect to throw junk into our mouths and think our bodies will respond kindly. No amount of fad supplements or even the latest fad super foods will help. Safe your money, time and energy.

The Alkaline Diet Lifestyle is not about dieting or eliminating your favorite foods forever. It's about adding more of the good and learning how to make better food choices. One more thing- there is no calorie counting on the alkaline diet.

Just eat clean and focus on alkaline foods. Ideally, about 70-80% of your diet should be comprised of alkaline foods. The recipes from this book, will help you be creative so that you can eat more alkaline. Go for a challenge. Try to have at least one alkaline smoothie a day.

Important: I am not saying that you should live on smoothies. This is not a smoothie cleanse book. Simply add more alkaline smoothies into your current diet as they will help you add in a ton of nutrients your body needs to pay you back with optimal wellbeing and abundant energy. The healthier you feel, the less unhealthy cravings you have. Health attracts health. Go for small changes. Baby steps.

Alkaline Foods are for you if:
- You've tried traditional "dieting" to lose weight and didn't like it
- You'd like to feel healthy and free of disease.
- You'd like to feel young and energetic again.
- You'd like to improve your skin.
- You'd like to stop being moody and irritated so often.
- You'd like to improve your concentration and digestion.

The book you are reading right now focuses on practical tips and smoothie recipes. Mostly, it is for those who have already been seasoned or have read my other books from the *Alkaline*

Diet Lifestyle Series. However, it also stands on its own. So, even if this is the first time you are hearing about the Alkaline Diet, diving into the recipes and reading all my additional tips, will give you the tools you need to start transforming your lifestyle today. No fluff, no theory, no complicated pH discussions; only effective solutions that work and are easy to apply even for busy individuals.

Additionally, I have 3 bonus PDF eBooks for you and a free VIP newsletter to help you keep on track. It will help you live and enjoy the alkaline diet. Even if you already follow an alkaline diet, it will give you more ideas for recipes and lifestyle tips:

www.holisticwellnessproject.com/alkaline

3 Free Bonus Guides

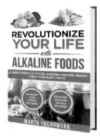 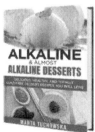 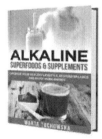

Problems with signing up? Email us:

info@holisticwellnessproject.com

Alkaline Smoothie Recipes-Recommended Shopping List

Opt for fresh and organic fruits and vegetables. Ordering items online may save time, or you may visit your local farmers' market. You can also order more and split with your neighbors and family to cut down costs. When it comes to fruits and vegetables, the fresher they are the better. You can also start growing your own.

ALKALINE INGREDIENTS

These ingredients are super alkaline. I suggest you make them your priority.

Here's the list of HIGH alkaline foods to use in your smoothies (this book will show you how to make it really delicious and fun!)

Alkaline Veggies:

- Beetroot
- Capsicum/Pepper
- Celery
- Chives
- Collard/Spring Greens
- Endive

- Garlic
- Ginger
- Lettuce
- Mustard Greens
- Okra
- Onion
- Radish
- Red Onion
- Rocket/Arugula
- Wakame seaweed
- Spinach and Kale
- Asparagus
- Carrot
- Courgette/Zucchini
- Leeks
- Pumpkin
- Squash
- Watercress
- Cucumber

These are NEUTRAL alkaline foods and can also be used in your smoothies:

- Cantaloupe
- Fresh Dates (in small amounts because they are rich in sugar)

- Nectarine
- Plum
- Sweet Cherry (Black Cherry)
- Watermelon
- Brazil Nuts
- Pecan Nuts
- Hazel Nuts
- Grapeseed Oil

Super Alkaline Fruits:

- Avocado
- Tomato
- Lemon
- Lime
- Grapefruit
- Fresh Coconut
- Pomegranate

Other Alkaline Smoothie Ingredients you might need:

- Herbal teas (cooled down)
- Herbs (basil, cinnamon, coriander, curry, rosemary, mint, thyme...)
- Almond milk
- Coconut water
- Coconut milk

OILS:

Don't forget about oils- these are "good oils":

- Avocado Oil
- Coconut Oil
- Flax Oil
- Udo's Oil
- Olive Oil

Alkaline nuts and seeds for more nutrients in your smoothies:

- Almonds
- Coconut
- Flax Seeds
- Pumpkin Seeds
- Sesame Seeds
- Sunflower Seeds

More recommendations:

- Filtered, preferably alkaline water (a simple water pitcher can be of great help)
- Himalayan salt -it contains magnesium, iron and other vital minerals and you can use it to give your smoothies and soups more taste.
- Grasses and quality powdered greens (you can have a look at my personal recommendations and extra resources at: www.HolisticWellnessProject.com/resources)
- Cucumber
- Kale
- Kelp
- Spinach (baby and grown)
- Parsley
- Broccoli
- All kinds of Sprouts (soy, alfalfa etc)
- Sea Vegetables (Kelp)

Understanding the Alkaline Diet (a simple, beginner-friendly explanation)

Now that we have gone through the food lists, you already intuitively understand what the alkaline diet is. So now, let's dive into details (it's not as complicated as some people make it to be, in fact, it's a very simple, balanced, common-sense healthy lifestyle).

According to the National Institute of Health, the pH of most of our crucial cellular and other body fluids like blood is designed to be at a pH of 7.365 which is slightly alkaline.

The body has an intricate system in place to maintain that healthy, slightly alkaline pH level no matter what you eat. This is an argument that many alkaline diet skeptics use, and I get it. It's 100% true, and I say the same thing.

This is not the goal of the alkaline diet. We just can't make our blood's pH more alkaline or "higher." Our body tries to work hard for us to help maintain our ideal pH.

We can't have a pH of 8 or 9. If we did, we would be dead. It's not about magically raising your pH (the main misconception about alkaline foods).

The focus of the alkaline diet is to give your body the nourishment and healing tools that it needs to MAINTAIN that optimal pH almost effortlessly.

If we fail to do so, we torture our body with incredible stress! Yes, when the body has to continually work overtime to detoxify all of the cells and maintain our pH, it finally succumbs to disease.

Let me name a few examples of what can happen if we continuously eat an acid-forming diet (also called SAD - Standard American Diet) and drink too much caffeine and sugar that does not support our body at all. Our body ends up sick and tired of working overtime and may manifest one or more of the following conditions:
- Constant inflammation and fat gain
- Immune and hormonal imbalance
- Lack of energy, mental fog- and you go for another cup of coffee yet still feel the same
- Yeast and candida overgrowth
- Digestive damage

- Weakened bones. Our body is forced to pull minerals like magnesium and calcium from our bones to maintain the alkaline balance it needs for constant healing processes.

In summary, eating more alkaline foods, for example veggies, herbs, and greens, helps support our body so that it can work for us at optimal levels while eating more acidic food (aka processed food, fast food etc.) doesn't help at all. The alkaline diet is not about magically raising our pH, but helping our body rebalance itself by supporting its natural healing functions.

Why is it called an alkaline diet, then?

To be honest, I don't know. It could also be called the Eat More Veggies diet, or perhaps Veggie Lover Diet, but then most people would never even look at it. I guess that it was called the alkaline diet for a reason, probably to make it more mysterious and sexy so that there is this "hook" that makes people think, "Hmmm, what is it? That stuff must be hot!".

Anyways...your body does not care what the name of this diet it. All it cares about is that you give it nutrient-dense foods so that it can pay you back with vibrant energy.

The alkaline diet is sisters with a clean food diet, anti-inflammatory diet, vegetarian diet, vegan diet, macrobiotic diet, and the raw food diet. In fact, it offers an incredible blend and the best of them all. All of those diets that are more in the plant-based diet category.

However, it's not only about what we eat. It's also about how we live and what we think. It's not just a diet; it's a lifestyle. If you want vibrant health and alkaline wellness, try to go outdoors more.

 Meditate, laugh, spend time with family and friends, do things you enjoy so that you can de-stress, and practice mindfulness. It's not only about nutrition. It's about your lifestyle. Again, this is exactly the message I share on my social media, my website and through my books.

A huge part of that lifestyle is also what we drink.

Set a simple, process-oriented goal to begin with. This strategy is what's proven to work for most people and personally I love focusing on process-oriented goals (while of course, making sure those goals align with my long-term health and wellness vision- for me it's constant transformation and taking others on that incredible journey too so that we can all empower and energize the planet!).

A process-oriented goal is for example when you decide to swap your afternoon coffee for a caffeine-free infusion. Or, create a morning or evening ritual where you enjoy a nice cup of alkaline tea, meditate, read or do something you enjoy. Just to spend some time with yourself and give yourself a well-deserved moment of reflection and meditation.

Whatever works for you, be my guest!

To sum up: The focus of the alkaline diet is to give your body the nourishment and the healing tools that it needs to MAINTAIN that optimal pH almost effortlessly.

This is achieved by taking in healthy, balanced nutrition rich in alkaline foods (you already know these are good for you!) such as:

- unprocessed foods
- naturally gluten-free foods
- yeast-free foods
- dairy-free foods
- sugar-free foods
- wheat-free foods
- foods rich in minerals, vitamins and chlorophyll
-plant-based foods, greens, herbs, spices and veggies

Now, you can easily determine what is or is not alkaline. Simple ask yourself:
-is it processed?
-does it contain gluten?
-does it contain dairy?
-does it contain sugar?
-is it rich in nutrients?

For example, lemons and limes are considered alkaline foods, because they are low in sugar and high in alkaline minerals (such as Magnesium).

Most fruit is not considered highly alkaline, because of higher sugar content. But...it's not about being perfect...

How to Create Balance on the Alkaline Diet

The reason I love the Alkaline Diet and found it much easier to implement and benefit from, is because of the alkaline 80/20 rule that most alkaline experts recommend. (It works so well!)

The rule is very simple. Your goal should be to make about 80% of your diet alkaline, while the remaining 20% can be other foods. Even 70/30 is a great start for most people.

It's as simple as making about three quarters of your plate full of alkaline foods, for example veggies. That allows for some flexibility as well as respect for other nutritional choices you may wish to combine with the Alkaline Diet. As far as the non-alkaline part of your diet is concerned, still try to make it as clean and healthy as possible. The 80/20 rule should not be interpreted as: 80% super healthy, alkaline and 20% some processed junk food (that would make your body go crazy).

The good news is that by enriching your diet with alkaline foods, automatically makes you crave more of good, healthy food (and less of unhealthy foods that take you away from your wellness goals).

Aside from working on your diet, I also recommend you start working on your lifestyle. Yes, you can enrich your lifestyle with more alkaline activities, such as relaxation, meditation and spending time in nature.

It's all interconnected.

If you want to explore self-care and self-love ideas, I warmly encourage you to check out my blog and my YouTube channel for extra tips, resources and inspiration:

www.HolisticWellnessProject.com/blog

www.HolisticWellnessProject.com/youtube

Amazing Alkaline Smoothie Recipes

Recipe Measurements

Personally, I am a big fan of making things easy. Life is already complicated enough. I love keeping ingredient measurements as simple as possible- this is why I stick to tablespoons, teaspoons and cups. You see, when it comes to making smoothies, you don't need to *be that precise*. What really matters is your time and simplicity.

The cup measurement I use is the American cup measurement. I also use it for dry ingredients. If you are new to it, let me help you:

If you don't have American Cup measures, just use a metric or imperial liquid measuring jug and fill your jug with your ingredient to the corresponding level. Here's how to go about it:

1 American Cup= 250ml= 8 fl.oz

For example:

If a recipe calls for 1 cup of almonds, simply place your almonds into your measuring jug until it reaches the 250 ml/8oz mark.

Quite easy, right?

I hope you found it helpful. I know that different countries use different measurements and I wanted to make things simple for you. I have also noticed that very often those who are used to American cup measurements complain about metric measurements and vice versa. However, if you apply what I have just explained, you will find it easy to use both.

Now, let's get busy blending...

Delicious Alkaline Smoothie Recipes

Green Exotic Blast for Massive Energy

You have probably heard the common recommendation preached by many health professionals- *have your 5 a day.* Well, the truth is that 5 a day may not be enough to help you create the balance and wellbeing you're seeking.

You see, 5 a day was probably enough 50 years ago when there was less pollution, less technology, more organic, clean food, and a healthier lifestyle. However, in this day and age, we need much more than just 5 a day, and this is what most alkaline diet experts encourage you to do.

So, imagine if you can get 7 or 8 a day- all at one time, in one delicious smoothie? Think of this wonderful, natural energy and how it will positively impact other areas of your life. Give yourself that energy, right here, right now.

Serves: 1-2

Ingredients:
- 1 cup coconut water (unsweetened)
- Half cup organic coconut cream (or thick coconut milk)
- Half avocado, peeled and pitted
- Half cup spinach
- Half cup of other leafy greens of your choice (for example kale)

- 1 cucumber, peeled and sliced
- 1 tablespoon basil
- 2 tablespoons coriander
- Juice of 1 lime
- 1 teaspoon of maca powder
- 1 teaspoon of chia seeds
- Pinch of chili powder
- Pinch of Himalayan salt
- Cup of filtered, preferably alkaline water (in case you don't want your smoothie too thick)

Instructions:
1. Blend cucumber, avocado, and greens; adding coconut water and coconut cream.
2. Now add the rest of the ingredients (basil, coriander, maca, chia seeds, chili powder, and Himalayan salt)

Additional Information

Is it worth going the extra mile to add some additional superfoods into your smoothie? Heck yea! Here is why...

Maca Powder

This natural supplement is rich in Vitamin C, B, and E, as well as zinc, iron, calcium, magnesium, phosphorus, and amino acids. It has hormone balancing properties and acts as an aphrodisiac both for men and women. As far as female health is concerned, maca can help alleviate menstrual cramps, as well as menopause issues (mood swings, depression, and anxiety).

Contraindications: avoid maca if pregnant or lactating. If on medication or suffering from any serious health problems, remember to contact your doctor first.

When trying maca for the first time, use no more than half teaspoon a day and go from there. The recommended maximum intake is actually about 1 teaspoon a day. However, remember that maca acts as a stimulant. Listen to your body, sometimes less is better.

Chia Seeds

Did you know that chia seeds contain more Omega-3s than salmon?

As a great source of fiber, protein, good fat, calcium, manganese, magnesium, phosphorus, as well as a good source of zinc, vitamin B3 (Niacin) Potassium, Vitamin B1, and Vitamin B2 (Thiamine), they really deserve the superfood badge. OK, so what are the benefits? To make it simple, chia seeds can help you:
-add more vital nutrients and antioxidants into your diet; hence, you will feel rejuvenated

-reduce or eliminate animal product consummation (chia seeds are an excellent from of protein for vegans and vegetarians)

-lose weight in a healthy way (they will help you embrace a healthier alkaline diet and feed your body with nutrients so you will crave less acidic foods that make you fat)

-have healthy bones and prevent osteoporosis (you already know it's a great source of calcium)

Now, your homework is to run to the nearest organic health store and buy some chia seeds or order online. You can thank me later!

Anti-Inflammatory Spicy Smoothie

When we add more nutritious alkaline meals, snacks, and smoothies into our diet, we help our body work for us in a more productive and efficient way. Our body is always looking for more and more, nutrient-dense, quality meals and drinks to pay us back with vibrant energy and wellbeing. This smoothie is a real treat- it's creamy, delicious and energizing!

I used to be a caffeine addict, and I needed a big cup of coffee in the afternoon. Otherwise, I couldn't keep going. Unfortunately, coffee and cow's milk, was making me even more sick and tired.

Developing this smoothie recipe was a real game changer for me. I gradually made it better and better by adding more alkaline-friendly ingredients as well as delicious spices to make it taste amazing!

Serves: 1-2
Ingredients:
- 1 tablespoon coconut oil
- 1-inch ginger root
- 1 teaspoon cinnamon (powder)
- 1 teaspoon cardamom (to infuse almond milk)
- 1 teaspoon nutmeg (to infuse almond milk)

- 1 bag rooibos tea (or about 10gr of loose rooibos leaves)
- 1 handful almonds (soaked in water for at least a few hours)
- 1 handful walnuts (soaked in water for at least a few hours)
- 1 tablespoon chia seeds
- 2 cups almond milk (unsweetened)
- Half avocado, peeled and pitted

Optional ingredients:

- 1 handful of kale or 1 tablespoon of green powders
- Half teaspoon of maca powder for more energy
- 1 teaspoon stevia to sweeten, if needed

Instructions:

1. First boil almond milk on medium heat.
2. When slightly boiling, add rooibos tea, cardamom, nutmeg, and ginger.
   My tip: you can always infuse more milk and store it in a fridge. It tastes delicious on its own, and you can do the same with coconut milk.
3. Now, let the spicy almond milk cool a bit.
4. When ready, strain and then place in a blender.
5. Add the main smoothie ingredients: avocado, nuts, and some green leaves.
6. Blend well until smooth.

7. Add some cinnamon powder and stevia (optional), coconut oil, chia seeds, and any additional ingredients of your choice (green powders or maca powder)
8. Serve slightly chilled.
9. Enjoy!

Additional Information:

The following ingredients will help you enjoy more energy and look glowing. Make sure you add them into your diet. They are natural superfoods, and the good news is that they are easy to get and will make your smoothies taste great.

-Kale, chia seeds, almond milk, and almonds are great sources of calcium. We were somehow brainwashed into thinking that we should drink milk to get our recommended dose of calcium, but...how did that work out? In our Western culture where drinking milk is, unfortunately, still a common thing to do, more and more people suffer from osteoporosis and other bone conditions and mineral deficiency. If, however, you compare this situation to many Asian countries where milk consumption is not practiced or not that widely practiced, you will see there are virtually no cases of osteoporosis. Take a look at a macrobiotic diet that originates from Japan. This diet is pretty alkaline and mostly plant-based in its design. There is no dairy. We don't need it. The problem with milk is that it is highly acidic, so it adds more acidity to our tissues, and our body, in order to seek balance, needs to keep depleting our bodies of calcium and other minerals. Vicious cycle. It's like asking for a loan with a really high interest rate. Something that is impossible to pay off. You then keep borrowing more and more money, only to end up in more debt. How efficient is it? How short-sighted is it?

Yet, we are still being brainwashed by TV commercials that milk and milk products are good for us...

Let me tell you this- those who decide to explore plant-based, sources of calcium and generally shift their diet in a more alkaline direction, report that they will never go back to drinking milk again. It would totally disagree with their stomach. Imagine you move from a really ugly and dangerous area to a nice and safe place, located in your favorite part of your town or city. Would you want to go back to where you lived before?

The problem is that, sometimes, people don't want to acknowledge the fact that they are not living but surviving. As soon as you discover the new alkaline, healthy world, you will leave the old, acidic world behind forever. Finally, you will start craving alkaline foods. Your taste buds will change!

-Coconut Oil: aside from its soft, exotic taste, it has plenty of health benefits. For example, it acts as a natural antimicrobial and helps clean the bacteria out of your esophagus.

-Finally, ginger possesses antioxidant and antimicrobial properties, and there is scientific proof that it helps combat reflux. According to the Journal of Molecular Nutrition & Food Research, it is actually eight times more effective at killing bacteria (the cause of acid reflux) than many standard medications.

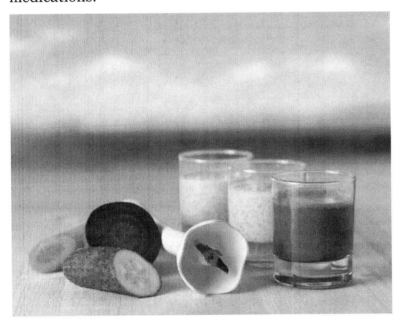

Easy Winter Smoothie

This smoothie is jam-packed with nutrients and will help boost your immune system. You can have it all year round; in the summer you can have it chilled with some ice-cubes, and in the winter you can heat it up a bit and have it as a thick soup.

Serves: 1-2

Ingredients:

- 3 tomatoes, peeled
- 1 celery stalk
- 2 cloves garlic, peeled
- 1-inch ginger, peeled
- 1 cucumber, peeled
- Juice of 1 lemon
- 1 cup filtered, preferably alkaline water (use less water if you want a thick, soup-like consistency)
- Pinch of Himalayan salt
- Pinch of black pepper
- Pinch of turmeric powder
- 1 tablespoon of olive oil, or avocado oil, or coconut oil, or udo's oil

Instructions:

1. Place tomatoes, celery, garlic, cucumber, and water in a blender and blend until smooth.
2. Add lemon juice, Himalayan salt, oil of your choice, black pepper, and turmeric.
3. Stir well.
4. Serve chilled or slightly warm and enjoy!

Additional Information:

-Start adding oils to your juices and smoothies. They will help your body absorb the nutrients. I usually use coconut oil (works great for exotic smoothies) and olive oil (I love it in vegetable smoothies and soups).

-The smoothie recipe I just presented to you is a great mix of alkaline power, nutrients, and vitamins that will help strengthen your immune system.

Here's a simple explanation:
Tomatoes are jam-packed with lycopene and antioxidants. Cucumbers are rich in lignans and phytonutrients that add to this smoothie's healing properties. Celery works as a natural anti-inflammatory, plus it's also full of Vitamin C, antioxidants, and flavonoids.

To sum up, I always say that there is no need to purchase exotic super foods and fruits with names you can't even pronounce. The best solutions are around us, and they can be acquired in a simple and inexpensive way.

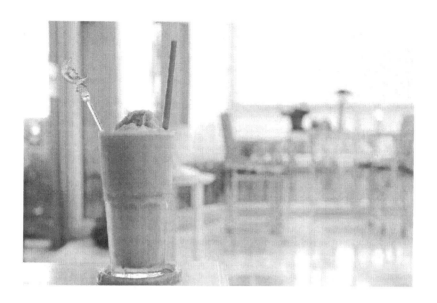

Liver Cleansing Smoothie

This original smoothie will help you get your high energy levels back. It's a great combination of alkaline and detoxifying ingredients, and its citric scent will help you energize your senses, as well.

This smoothie will be more effective if you consume it first thing in the morning before you have eaten anything.

Serves: 1- 2
Ingredients:

- 2 grapefruits, juiced (you can use a simple lemon squeezer)
- 2 lemons, juiced (a simple lemon squeezer will do)
- Half cup water, filtered, preferably alkaline
- 2 tablespoons of flax oil or olive oil
- 2 cucumbers, peeled
- 1 avocado, peeled and pitted
- 2 cloves of fresh garlic, peeled
- 1-inch ginger
- Pinch of Himalayan salt
- Pinch of cayenne pepper

Instructions:

1. In a blender, combine cucumber, garlic, ginger, and avocado with some lemon and grapefruit juice.

2. Blend until smooth.
3. Add alkaline water, oil, and spices.
4. Stir well and drink to your health.
5. Enjoy!

Additional Information

So, what makes this smoothie so effective in taking care of your liver?

-Garlic is rich in sulfur-containing compounds that stimulate the liver enzymes responsible for getting rid of toxins from the body. It is also rich in other important nutrients, such as allicin and selenium, which help protect your liver. It has anti-cancer properties, helps prevent fatty liver, and lower cholesterol levels. Of course, don't overdo garlic. You don't want those around you to start avoiding you, right?

Fortunately, grapefruit juice from this recipe helps neutralize garlic's odor. So... nothing to worry about!

-Ginger: just like garlic, it helps to prevent liver damage and works as a natural antioxidant. It also stimulates digestion.

-Grapefruit: this alkaline fruit contains limonoids that stimulate massive production of a super powerful detoxifying enzyme called glutathione-S-transferase. This enzyme helps your liver remove more toxins.

-Lemons: they contain limonoids so they help support liver function, stimulating a detoxification process.

-Omega 3: (flax oil is rich in Omega 3) is a powerful anti-inflammatory agent that helps take care of your liver and kidneys.

Overall, this smoothie offers a great combination of taste and liver-healing ingredients!

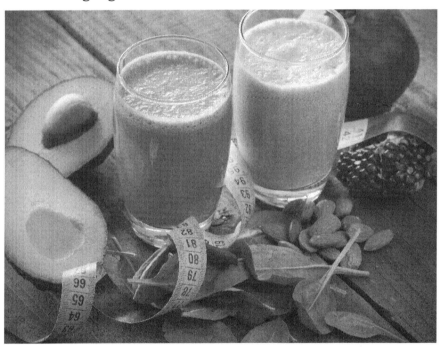

Vitamin C Power Fruity Smoothie

This smoothie tastes and smells delicious. It will re-energize your body and mind in a few seconds.

Vitamin C is crucial for proper iron absorption, as well as taking care of your immune system, cardiovascular system, collagen synthesis, and antioxidant activities.

Trust me, there is no need to resort to that many supplements if you take care of your diet first.

Serves: 2

Ingredients:

- 1 cup almond milk or coconut milk (raw, unsweetened)
- 1 grapefruit, peeled
- 1 kiwi, peeled
- 1 avocado, peeled and pitted
- 1 green apple, cut in smaller pieces
- A few leaves of fresh mint
- Optional: stevia to sweeten if needed

Instructions:

1. Place all the ingredients in a blender.
2. Blend well until smooth.

3. If you are new to smoothies or like them sweeter, add some natural stevia powder. Avoid commercial versions of stevia that are full of chemicals.

4. Enjoy!

Additional Information

Very often, I get asked about fruit on the alkaline diet. I see that many people get paranoid about fruit. But the alkaline rule is actually really simple; you are encouraged to focus on non-sugary, alkaline fruits like limes, lemons, pomegranates, grapefruits, etc.

Avocados and tomatoes are also highly alkalizing fruits. The rest of the fruits are usually considered to be neutral or mildly acid-forming because of their high sugar content. What I always advise people to do is to listen to their body and observe their digestion.

Personally, I like fruit in moderate amounts, especially in the summer, but too much fruit does not agree with my stomach. I also use non-alkaline fruits, like bananas (these are not considered super alkaline because of their high sugar content), because they are my favorite super food, and they provide me with energy (again- balance and moderation are the key).

To sum up, if you ask me about fruit, I am in the middle of the road. I am not getting too paranoid about them, but at the same time, I do not preach that all fruits have super alkalizing properties (most of them don't). I am a big proponent of balance, and this is what I try to achieve with my nutrition, as well. As you can see, in my smoothies, I focus mostly on alkaline and super alkaline ingredients; however, I do not steer clear of other fruits. I like variety.

Remember the 80/ 20 rule (70/30 is also fine). Focus on alkaline foods first (the bigger part of your diet). Fruit is OK in your 20-30%. There is no reason to eliminate it at all.

If you want to learn more about alkaline vs acidic foods, don't forget to sign up for your 3 free PDF guides with detailed charts and email updates to help you stay on track. www.HolisticWellnessProject.com/alkaline

Moderately Alkaline Strawberry Summer Smoothie

Coconut water is one of my healthy addictions. I love it in my smoothies. It has an amazing, exotic flavor and is jam-packed with nutrients like potassium, calcium, iron, manganese, magnesium, and zinc. It is also a good source of B-complex vitamins such as riboflavin, niacin, thiamin, pyridoxine, and folates.

Alkalinity and hydration go hand in hand, and coconut water provides optimal hydration. If you are interested in weight loss smoothies, use coconut water as your smoothie base. It will give your body what it needs to start losing weight naturally; it will help rebalance your pH, detoxify your body, provide your body with vital nutrients, and satisfy your sweet tooth.

Serves: 2
Ingredients:
- Half cup organic strawberries
- 2 cups coconut water
- Half inch ginger, peeled
- 2 grapefruits, peeled
- 2 tablespoons hemp seed or chia seed powder

Instructions:

1. Place in a blender and blend until smooth.

2. Serve with some ice cubes.

3. Enjoy!

Additional Information and Tips

Ginger is miraculous and super alkalizing. I love making ginger ice cubes. Simply juice as much ginger as you can, mix with some water, and freeze into ice cubes. These will always be ready to grab and use with your smoothies, fruit infused water, teas, and other drinks.

Quick Energy Boost Smoothie

Let me be honest with you. We are just about to do some cheating. Why? Well, it's simple: all forms of caffeine are acid-forming. This is why caffeinated drinks are usually off the alkaline diet.

However, as an ex-caffeine addict, I know that it's not easy to transition from hectoliters of coffee to green smoothies. Very few people can go cold turkey even if, deep inside, they want to. It's because of the fact that when your body gets addicted to caffeine, it starts suffering from side effects, like headaches or even moodiness, when you just "switch it off" from one day to another.

I also believe that there is nothing wrong with an occasional use of caffeine. Personally, I am a big fan of green tea. Of course, don't overdo it. This is why I recommend you try this smoothie. It will help you make a transition. Besides, green tea is also full of antioxidants. Whether you are trying to quit, reduce caffeine, do it step-by-step, or just get on a "controlled" caffeine high, this is the recipe for you to try.

Notice how alkaline ingredients can help achieve balance! This is what it's all about.

Serves: 2

Ingredients:

- 1 cup of green tea, cooled down (use 1 tea bag or 1 teaspoon of green tea per cup)
- 1 grapefruit, juiced (a simple lemon squeezer will do)
- 1 cup pomegranates
- 1 green apple, seeds removed
- Optional: stevia to sweeten
- A few slices of limes or lemons to garnish

Instructions:

1. Place in a blender.
2. Blend well until smooth.
3. Enjoy!

Additional Information

While I always say that you don't need to depend on caffeine for energy (this is why I am writing this book; I want to show you how you can do it with raw and alkaline foods in the form of delicious smoothies), I really like green tea, and personally, I think it's a good addition to a balanced, alkaline diet (even though green tea is not alkaline, the alkaline lifestyle is not about sticking to 100% alkaline ingredients. It's all about balance!).

Let's have a look at some of the benefits of green tea:

-Better focus, concentration, and mental alertness: green tea has less caffeine than coffee, which is a good thing, as too much caffeine results in an energy clash. However, this benefit is not so much due to caffeine presence in green tea, but more because it is rich in a substance called L-theanine.

According to the Journal of Nutrition, L-theanine is an amino-acid that can increase the activity of the inhibitory neurotransmitter, GABA, which has anti-anxiety effects. Aside from that, it also helps release more dopamine (natural high!) and produce alpha waves in the brain (better concentration). L-theanine works in synergy with caffeine and has been proven effective in bettering brain function.

-fat burn and improved metabolic rate

-natural anti-cancer drink: according to numerous studies, green tea has powerful antioxidants that may protect against different kinds of cancer.

-less infection and better dental health- the catechins in green tea can prevent the growth of bacteria and some viruses responsible for caries, bad breath, and infections.

To sum up, if you need some caffeine in your life, green tea is a great drink to turn to. Of course, moderation is the key.

Minty Refreshment with an Alkaline Twist

This is one of my favorite summer smoothies. I invented it by accident. You see, I ran out of plant-based milks, and I think that using water in smoothies is somewhat boring.

I was looking for another liquid that is healthy, alkaline, and refreshing, and I realized that I had lots of fresh mint.

I decided to go overboard and prepared a really strong mint infusion. Then, I just blended in a few ingredients I had on-hand and was pretty impressed by the result.

Serves: 2

Ingredients:

- 2 cups of mint tea (use 2-4 tea bags per 2 cups of water)
- 1 cucumber, peeled
- 2 green apples, seeds removed
- Half cup blueberries
- Optional: stevia to sweeten
- A few slices of lime or lemon to garnish.

Instructions:

1. Blend until smooth.
2. Add some ice cubes and sweeten with stevia, according to your personal preferences.
3. Garnish with lime or lemon slices.
4. Drink to your health and enjoy!

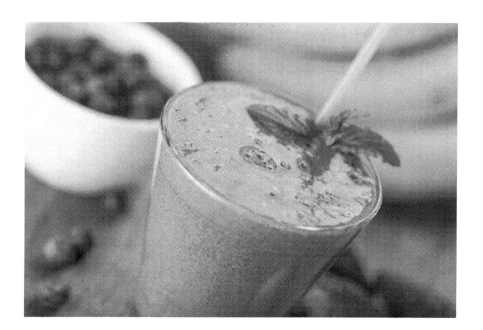

Simple Super Alkaline Powerfoods Smoothie

I love cucumbers. They are easy to get, refreshing, and packed with nutrients. In other words, they are one of my favorite alkaline super foods. They are full of vital minerals and nutrients like Vitamin A, Pantothenic Acid, Magnesium, Phosphorus, Manganese, Vitamin C, Vitamin K, and Potassium.

Cucumber is also a fantastic ingredient in natural beauty treatments. Don't throw away those cucumber peels; use them to refresh your skin. This is especially recommended for oily and mixed complexions or after sunbathing.

Serves: 2
Ingredients:
- 2 cucumbers, peeled
- 2 grapefruits, peeled
- 2 cups coconut milk (raw, unsweetened)
- 1 tablespoon of raisins
- 2 tablespoons almond powder (or almonds)
- 2 lemons, juiced
- Cinnamon and ginger powder (optional)
- A few mint leaves to garnish

Instructions:

1. Blend the cucumbers, grapefruits, and raisins with coconut milk.
2. Mix well. Now, add some almond powder, spices, and lemon juice.
3. Stir well again.
4. Garnish with some mint leaves.
5. Serve with some ginger ice cubes for optimal wellbeing.
6. Enjoy!

Cherried Beet Smoothie

To be quite honest with you, I don't really like beets. However, I am aware of their nutritional value. They are packed with calcium, iron, vitamins A and C, folic acid, fiber, manganese, and potassium. I also knew they were super alkalizing. This is why I decided to experiment and create a beet smoothie that is extremely refreshing and delicious.

This is my tip for you- think of alkaline foods that you can't imagine eating on their own. For some of you, my dear readers, it can be kale or spinach; for some it may be broccoli or beets or something else. The next step is to mix them with some alkaline fruits or veggies you like so that you can enjoy all their nutrients, but at the same time, create a delicious recipe.

There is always a way to make a delicious smoothie, even if one of its ingredients is not on your favorite foods list.

Serves: 2

Ingredients:

- Half cup cherries, pitted
- Half cup beets
- 1 cup water (filtered, alkaline)
- 1 cup coconut milk
- 1 tablespoon coconut oil
- Pinch of organic vanilla powder and cinnamon
- Pinch of stevia (optional)
- A few mint leaves and lime slices to garnish

Instructions:

1. Combine berries, beets, banana slices, water, and coconut milk in a blender.
2. Blend until smooth. If you like it creamy, then don't use water; add more coconut milk instead.
3. Mix in some coconut oil, vanilla, and cinnamon. If you like it sweet, then add some stevia too.
4. Garnish with mint leaves and lime slices.
5. Serve and enjoy!

Additional Information

Naturopathic doctors recommend beets as a natural medicine for many conditions including liver disorders, constipation, high cholesterol, and immune system disorders. Beets are also great juiced. For more nutritional benefits, you can juice beets with the leaves and have this juice with some lemon juice and olive oil. This will work as a shot of health and a natural liver cleanser.

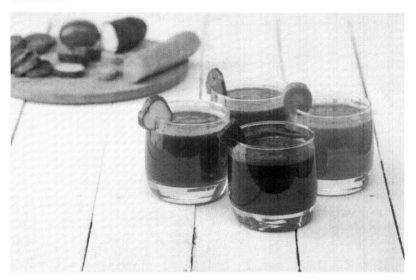

Simple Kale Smoothie

Here comes another simple smoothie recipe that will make adding more greens into your diet painless and easy.

Kale is one of the alkaline super foods. It is highly alkalizing and a great source of dietary fiber, protein, thiamin, riboflavin, folate, iron, magnesium, and phosphorus.

It is also rich in vitamin A, vitamin C, vitamin K, vitamin B6, calcium, potassium, copper, and manganese. Give your body the optimal body and mind energy it deserves!

Serves: 2
Ingredients:
- 1 cup kale leaves
- 2 pears, peeled and cut into smaller pieces
- 1 cup water, filtered, preferably alkaline
- 2 lemons, juiced (a simple lemon squeezer will do)
- 2 tablespoons coconut oil
- Optional: stevia to sweeten

Instructions:

1. Combine water, lemon juice, kale, and pears in a blender.
2. Blend until smooth.
3. Now, add some coconut oil (liquefied) and stevia, if you like it sweet.
4. Stir well.
5. Serve and enjoy!

Easy Antioxidant Fat Burn Smoothie

Have you ever tried Chinese Pu-Erh tea? Did you know that it has fat burning properties? It is also helps reduce cholesterol and improve mental alertness. It contains much less caffeine than coffee or black tea, but since it's not totally caffeine-free, so avoid it if you are caffeine intolerant, pregnant, lactating, or if you suffer from any medical conditions that require a 100% caffeine-free lifestyle.

If this is your case, then replace pu-Erh tea from this recipe with an herbal, caffeine-free infusion that is safe to take in your condition or use coconut water instead. Still, drinking pu-erh tea in moderate amounts is safe.

I am in the habit of having 1 cup of pu-erh tea a day, or I use it with my smoothies. Usually, in the winter, I like warm teas with ginger and lemon juice; however, in the summer, I like using teas and cold infusions, smoothies, or fruit infused water.

I especially recommend this smoothie if you are wanting to lose weight and burn fat.

Serves: 2

Ingredients:

- 1 cup of pu-erh tea, cooled
- 1 cup almond milk (unsweetened)
- A few pineapple slices (optional)
- Half cup blueberries
- 1 big grapefruit, peeled
- A handful of spinach leaves
- Optional: stevia to sweeten

Instructions:

1. Place all the ingredients in a blender.
2. Blend until smooth.
3. Add some stevia to sweeten and ice cubes, if you like it cool. I especially recommend ginger ice cubes. They will add to this smoothie's detoxifying properties.
4. Enjoy and let the red tea smoothie work for you and your body!

Kukicha Smoothie

Ever heard of kukicha? If not, make sure you put it on your alkaline shopping list. If yes, I hope the following recipe will help you come up with more ideas on your alkaline journey. Kukicha tea has been commonly used in Chinese and Japanese Natural Medicine to fight:

•   Digestion problems and constipation

•   Bladder infections

•   Low energy levels

•   High cholesterol and high blood pressure

•   Cancer

•   Excess weight (Kukicha tea helps detoxify and alkalize the body)

Serves: 2

Ingredients:

- 1 cup kukicha tea, cooled down
- 1 cup coconut milk
- Half cup spinach
- 1 small banana, peeled
- 1-inch ginger, peeled
- 1-inch turmeric, peeled
- A handful of almonds (soaked in water for 8 hours or more)
- Optional: juice of 1 lemon

Instructions:

1. Blend all the ingredients until smooth.
2. Add some lemon juice to spice it up (and add some Vitamin C).
3. Stir well, serve, and enjoy!

Additional Information

Do you know what excessive caffeine intake does to your body? Well, it depletes it of iron, magnesium, and other minerals that your body needs, not only to maintain a healthy pH, but also for healthy bones and tissues.

I have already said that, personally, I think there is nothing wrong with enjoying a nice cup of organic coffee, black tea, or green tea every now and then. The problem is if the "every now and then" becomes an addiction, and you need to depend on hectoliters of caffeinated drinks of all kinds to keep you going. Kukicha can help you make a transition.

It's virtually caffeine-free and full of zinc, iron, selenium, copper, manganese, fluoride, B vitamins, Vitamin A, Theanine, amino acids, and flavanoids.

It tastes amazingly delicious with almond milk, gluten-free rice milk (not compatible with Paleo diets, though), or coconut milk. You may sweeten it with some stevia.

In the winter, I like it with some lemon or grapefruit juice. Make sure you add the juice when your tea is not boiling but slightly warm. That way, you make sure you don't kill the vitamins from your juice. After all, this is why we want it, right?

To sum up- if you want to increase your energy levels, reduce caffeine intake, feel rejuvenated, and have beautiful skin, resort to kukicha tea. You can thank me later!

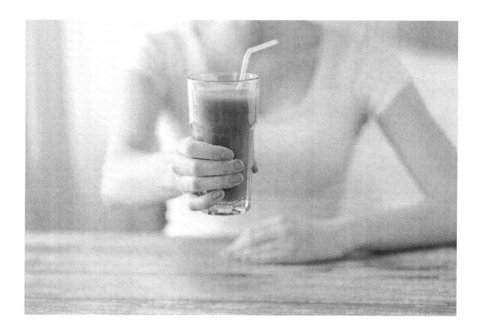

Original Veggie Smoothie

Ok, I know that some of my readers won't like this recipe. I know it may seem strange at first. But please, read with an open mind. The problem is that our society has mostly conditioned us to think of smoothies as ice-creamy fruity treats (very often with sugar, milk and dairy products as main ingredients). This is why some of us may think it's kind of weird to use green veggies as smoothie ingredients!

I encourage you to think of this smoothie as a creamy soup or a vegetable cream. It will help you add more greens into your diet, and this is one of our alkaline diet goals, right?

Serves: 2
Ingredients:
- 1 cup broccoli, steamed
- 1 bunch asparagus, steamed
- 2 cups coconut milk
- 2 tablespoons coconut oil
- 2 carrots, peeled
- A few inches of horseradish
- Himalayan salt
- Pinch of chili powder
- A few onion rings
- 2 garlic cloves, peeled

Instructions:

1 Place all ingredients except coconut oil, chili powder, and salt in a blender.

2 Blend well until smooth.

3 Mix in some Himalayan salt, coconut oil, and chili powder.

4 Stir well and serve!

5 You can have it chilled (great in hot summers) or slightly warm. If you go for the second option, remember not to overdo the heating. Try not to exceed 100 Fahrenheit (around 35 Celsius) so as to keep the vital nutrients.

Additional information:

Recently, I have really taken to horseradish. I love it in my salads (usually spiralized), stir-fries, curry dishes, creams, soups, and smoothies. Horseradish adds intriguing taste and flavor. It is also inexpensive. There we go again!

We have another common-sense alkaline food to add to our alkaline shopping list.

Have a look at the health benefits and decide for yourself:

- Horseradish is rich in dietary fiber, vitamins, minerals, and antioxidants.

- It works as a natural anti-inflammatory and diuretic.

- It is rich in vitamin-C, helps boost immunity, and gets rid of dangerous free-radicals from your body

- It also contains minerals like sodium, potassium, manganese, iron, copper, zinc, magnesium, as well as, essential vitamins such as folate, vitamin B-6, riboflavin, niacin, and pantothenic acid.

Nice'n Fresh Smoothie

Soy sprouts and alfalfa sprouts are great, not only in your salads and soups, but also in your smoothies. When combined with other healthy and alkalizing ingredients, they create amazing alkaline balance and taste.

Serves: 2

Ingredients:

- 2 cups almond milk (unsweetened)
- Half cup soy sprouts
- Half cup alfalfa sprouts
- 1-inch ginger, peeled
- Half avocado, peeled and pitted
- 1 green apple, seeds removed
- 1 tablespoon avocado oil or coconut oil
- stevia to sweeten (optional)

Instructions:

1. Combine all the ingredients, except for oils, in a blender.
2. Blend until smooth.
3. Add some coconut oil or avocado oil. If you wish, sweeten with some stevia.
4. Enjoy!

Additional Information:

The benefits of avocado oil:

- It is a great source of Vitamin E and has anti-ageing properties.
- It is a great source of protein and unsaturated fats.
- It is rich in antioxidants.

While avocado oil is not a must-have ingredient (you can stick to olive oil and coconut oil, instead), I encourage you to learn more about it, and whenever you get a chance, try it. I used to stick too closely to olive oil and refused to leave my comfort zone. I finally decided to enrich my diet with other oils so as not to get bored. Again, I could have done well without it, but I believe that real health (and life) success is about constant learning and exploring. This is what you are doing now as you are reading this book!

Now, let's move on to the next alkaline recipe …

Lemon Smoothie Refreshment

You already know that Alkalinity and hydration go hand in hand. If you find water too boring, go for hydrating and nourishing fruits like melons (cantaloupe). They taste great in smoothies, especially when combined with some ice cubes.

This is one of my latest summer smoothie recipes. Great taste, hydration, and Alkalinity are combined. Yes, you can have it all; you deserve unstoppable energy and vibrant health.

Serves: 2
Ingredients:
- 2 cups coconut or almond milk
- Half cup melon, chopped
- Half avocado, peeled and pitted
- Half cucumber, peeled and sliced
- Ice cubes (I recommend you make ginger ice cubes for more taste and optimal wellbeing)
- 2 limes, juiced (a simple lemon squeezer will do)
- 1 tablespoon coconut oil, liquefied

Instructions:

1. Place all the ingredients except coconut oil in a blender.
2. Blend until smooth and add some coconut oil.
3. Stir well.
4. Enjoy the freshness!

Additional Information:

Melons are a great source of niacin, fiber, Vitamin B6, folate, as well as, Vitamin A, Vitamin C, and Potassium. They are not super alkalizing, as they do not belong to non-sugary fruit, but they are not super acidifying either.

They fall in the middle of alkaline-acid charts and can be described as neutral. Personally, I can't imagine summers without melons. I also use them to make lemonades and fruit-infused water.

Sweet Dreams Smoothie

You already know that I am a big fan of herbal infusions and that I also like to use them in my smoothies. After all, if it's always coconut milk or almond milk, it may get a bit boring, right? Besides, herbal infusions have unique healing properties.

For example, Melissa helps soothe the nerves, stimulate digestion, and sleep better. This smoothie has an amazing taste and is very refreshing. I recommend it as an evening treat that will help you unwind... Oat milk mixes really well with this smoothie, as it also has sleep inducing properties. Make sure to go for organic, gluten-free oat milk.

Serves: 2
Ingredients:
- 1 cup Melissa infusion, chilled (if making this smoothie for 2 people, use 2 tea bags)
- 1 cup oat milk, unsweetened, organic, gluten-free (if you follow a Paleo diet, choose almond or coconut milk instead)
- A handful of cherries, pitted (you can also use blueberries instead)
- 1-inch ginger
- 1-inch turmeric

- 1 cup pomegranates

Instructions:

1. Place all the ingredients in a blender.
2. Blend well until smooth.
3. Use stevia to sweeten, if you wish, and add some ice cubes for extra refreshment.
4. Enjoy!

Additional Information

The healing properties of Melissa (Lemon balm):

-Helps fight insomnia and provides deep relaxation

-Caffeine-free

-Reduces pain (menstrual cramps, headache)

-Can help improve your mood

Precautions: while some resources say it is safe in pregnancy, other say it is not. I suggest you remain on the safe side and avoid it when pregnant (unless your herbalist and doctor state otherwise). It is not recommended to use when a person is on medical tranquilizing drugs; it may interact with CNS depressants. If overdosed, Melissa may cause dizziness and sleepiness (abstain from driving).

Sweet Dreams Smoothie 2

This is a variation of a previous smoothie for those of you who wish to try more herbs or simply don't like Melissa, for some reason. You could also mix Melissa and verbena together. It's up to you.

Serves: 2

Ingredients:

- 1 cup verbena tea (use 1 teabag per cup)
- 1 cup almond or coconut milk
- Half cup blueberries
- 1 small avocado, peeled and pitted
- Half inch ginger, peeled
- Half teaspoon cinnamon powder

Instructions:

1. Place all the ingredients in a blender.
2. Blend until smooth.
3. Enjoy!

Additional Information

The Benefits of Verbena:

-improves digestion

-strengthens the nervous system and the immune system

-gives relief in fever, colds, and flu

-stimulates relaxation and better sleep

-Reduces PMS

Verbena is a safe herb, but there is not enough information to confirm whether it can be used during pregnancy or breast-feeding. The same applies to possible contraindications with other medications. I always recommend consulting with your doctor first.

Extra information:

Have you ever tried verbena essential oil? It is miraculous! It is definitely one of my favorite oils and a great natural way to help you relax and enjoy better sleep. I usually use it for self-massage. I mix a few drops in a tablespoon of coconut oil or other vegetable oil, and I massage my neck, shoulders, and feet. Verbena essential oil smells phenomenal...It's a great way to unwind and create your holistic spa at home.

Relaxation Digestion and Better Sleep Smoothie

Relaxation, digestion, and better sleep ... 3 in 1 smoothie? Sound too good to be truth? Well, good things exist, and you deserve them. You can say thanks to fennel.

It is an amazing herb with a myriad of properties. Its natural, sweet taste is a great component of herbal, alkaline smoothies.

Serves: 2

Ingredients

- 1 cup fennel tea infusion (use 2 teabags if serving 2 people), cooled down
- 1 cup almond milk
- 1 cup watermelon, chopped
- Half cup pomegranates
- 1-inch ginger, peeled
- 1-inch turmeric, peeled

Instructions:

1. Place all the ingredients in a blender.
2. Blend until smooth.
3. Enjoy!

Additional Information

The healing benefits of fennel tea:

-reduces bloating and flatulence

-great in natural anti-cellulite treatments

-soothes colds and flu

-has anti-inflammatory properties and is recommended for those suffering from joint pain and arthritis

-acts as a natural antioxidant and alkalizes the blood

Caution:

Since fennel tea lowers the blood pressure, consult with your doctor if you are on any blood pressure medication. In case of any serious health problems or if on any medication, you should consult with your doctor first, even if choosing natural herbal options.

Many herbs may interact with certain pharmaceutical drugs, and it's always better to stay on the safe side.

If you are looking to get rid of a specific condition and use natural herbal treatments, it is always advised to consult a naturopathic doctor for better results (this is what I do when I need to "fix myself").

What is your favorite recipe so far? If you have a few seconds please let me know in the review section of this book. I would love to hear from you!

Beautiful Skin Alkaline Smoothie

Here comes a really simple and effective smoothie recipe for beautiful skin and a better, healthy- looking tan. It is a must-drink in the summer!

Serves: 2

Ingredients:

- 1 grapefruit, peeled
- 1 cup coconut water
- 3 carrots, peeled
- 3 tomatoes, peeled
- 1-inch turmeric, peeled

Instructions:

1. Blend all the ingredients in a blender until smooth.
2. Drink to your beauty and health!
3. Enjoy!

Additional Information

What's the point of swallowing Vitamin A pills if there is a better, healthier, more natural way? Moreover, it can be done in an inexpensive way. Carrots are another common-sense super food! Personally, I love carrots as a snack with vegetable-herbal dips, hummus, or guacamole. Yummy and healthy!

Health benefits of carrots:

- Helps cleanse the body as it is rich in Vitamin A, which aids the liver in getting rid of toxins from the body.

-Better vision (say thanks to Vitamin A again!)

-Natural anti-age and antioxidant, as it is rich in beta-carotene

-Healthy skin, nails, and hair. Prevents premature wrinkling as well as acne

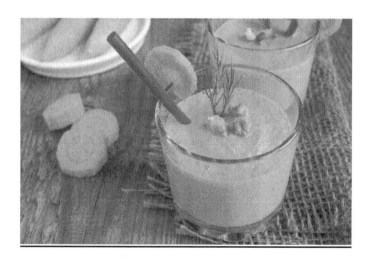

White Dream Energy Smoothie

After getting started on alkaline smoothies, you will soon realize that creativity and constant experiments are the key to success. Many people quit, as they get bored with the same smoothie or the same ingredients.

My tip is always to try to experiment with different kinds of plant based and nut milks. The most alkaline would be coconut milk and almond milk, and these are my favorite (check the bonus recipe at the back end of this book to check how to make your own). However, there are many other options out there. One of them is hazelnut milk! So yummy!

Serves: 2
Ingredients:
- 2 cups hazelnut milk
- 1 cup shredded coconut
- A few banana slices
- Half avocado, peeled and sliced
- A handful of spinach leaves, washed
- Juice of 2 limes
- 2 cinnamon sticks
- Optional: ice cubes

Instructions:

1. Place all the ingredients in a blender.
2. Blend until smooth.
3. Infuse with cinnamon sticks for a couple of hours (better to store your smoothie in a fridge).
4. Drink to your health!

Additional Information

The benefits of hazelnut milk:

-improved mental focus and more energy, as it is a good source of vitamins B1, B2, and B6

-healthy hair and skin, as it is rich in Vitamin E

-natural source of protein

-helps control cholesterol levels, as it is rich in omega-3 fatty acid ALA

Plus... it tastes delicious. I love the nutty flavor. You can use it to make healthy pancakes and desserts!

Easy Natural Protein Smoothie

Have you ever tried to add quinoa to your smoothies? If not, the time is now. Don't worry about the "all grains are bad for you" thing. You see, quinoa is a good grain, and it's gluten-free. Heck, I even know some Paleo people who make an exception and eat quinoa, as they know how healthy it is. So even if you are Paleo, try this recipe.

Serves: 2

Ingredients:

- Half cup quinoa, cooked
- 1 tablespoon hemp seed powder
- 2 cups hazelnut milk
- A handful of kale leaves, washed
- Juice of 2 limes
- Half cup pomegranates
- A few banana slices
- Stevia to sweeten, if needed

Instructions:

1. Place all the ingredients in a blender and blend until smooth.
2. Stir well to make sure there are no lumps.
3. Enjoy and drink to your energy and health!

Additional Information

If you want to learn why you should get hooked on quinoa, check out my article:

www.holisticwellnessproject.com/quinoa

It will also give you a few extra recipe ideas to help you on your journey.

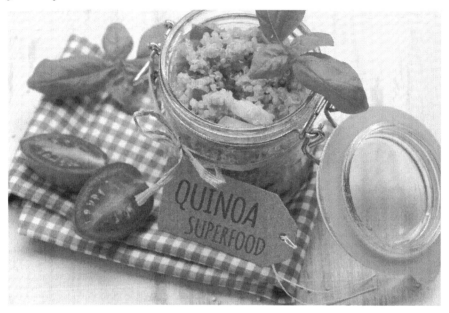

Simple Apple Cucumber Smoothie

Sometimes, all you need is simplicity, and this is what this smoothie offers. Personally, I love combining cucumbers with apples. This is how I create balance. If you have downloaded the alkaline-acid charts from my free guide (www.HolisticWellnessProject.com/alkaline), you have probably noticed that cucumbers are highly alkaline, whereas apples are moderately acidic. However, the alkalinity of cumbers and coconut milk, as well as, spices and Himalayan salt, outweigh the slight acidity of apples.

Remember about the 80/20 rule. The alkaline diet is not about sticking to 100% alkaline green foods. We are not rabbits.

Just seek to make about 80% of your diet alkaline. Many alkaline diet experts say that even 70% alkaline is enough. This is not a difficult goal to achieve. Also, not all acidic foods are bad. For example, apples are a great source of Vitamin C, antioxidants, and dietary fiber and a great part of a balanced, alkaline diet.

Serves: 2
Ingredients:
- 1 green apple, seeded
- 2 cucumbers, peeled

- 1 cup almond milk
- Half cup coconut cream (raw, organic)
- Pinch of cinnamon and nutmeg
- Pinch of Himalayan salt
- 1 tablespoon coconut oil

Instructions:

1. Place all the ingredients in a blender and blend until smooth.
2. Mix in some coconut oil, spices, and Himalayan salt.
3. Enjoy!

Additional Information

If you want to create a new, healthy habit that will only take a few seconds, make sure you add some cinnamon and nutmeg to your smoothies. You can get them in powder, ready to mix in.

Both cinnamon and nutmeg have strong anti-inflammatory properties and will add to the alkalizing benefits of your smoothies.

Hormone Rebalancer Natural Energy Smoothie

This smoothie recipe is a fantastic option if you don't like green smoothies, but you still want to experience all the health benefits of alkaline smoothies.

It's very easy to make, tastes delicious and is jam-packed with nutrients.

Servings: 1-2

Ingredients:

- 1 big grapefruit, peeled and halved
- 1 cup water (filtered, preferably alkaline)
- 1 inch of ginger, peeled
- 1 tablespoon coconut oil
- Half teaspoon maca powder
- Stevia to sweeten, if desired

Instructions:

1. Blend all the ingredients in a blender.
2. Serve and enjoy!

Green Mineral Comfort Smoothie Soup

This recipe can be used both as a smoothie as well as a "smoothie style soup".

It's very easy to make and great as a side dish, or a quick detox meal.

Servings: 1-2

Ingredients:

- 1 big cucumber, peeled
- 1 small avocado, peeled and pitted
- 1 carrot, peeled
- A handful of cilantro
- 1 cup of thick coconut milk
- A handful of raw almonds
- 1 tablespoon of olive oil
- Himalayan salt to taste
- 1 small chili flake (if you like it spicy)

Instructions:

1. Blend all the ingredients in a blender.
2. Serve as a smoothie, or as a soup (raw or lightly cooked).
3. Enjoy!

BONUS RECIPES: How to Make Almond Milk and Coconut Milk

Raw Almond Milk

Of all plant-based milk we can create, almond milk is certainly my favorite. Personally, I am not a big fan of soy milk, because large amounts don't agree with my stomach (even though I have always stuck to organic options).

I have also experimented with rice milk, but I finally discovered an even more natural, nutritious, and raw (aside from coconut milk that I always praise) is raw almond milk.

You can make your own and save money. Besides, if you make your own, you always know its ingredients. I remember looking for almond milk in bio supermarkets and in organic stores where I live. To my disappointment, most of them had added sugar (even though they had an "organic" label on them), and those that didn't were extremely expensive.

This predicament has driven me to create my own rituals and make my own almond milk. Try it yourself! Almond milk is also Paleo-friendly (for those of you who follow Paleo) while soy milk and rice milk aren't. Still, when I was starting on my dairy-free journey, I would try different options to see what worked for me. Lesson learned- almond milk rocks!

After you have created this recipe, store your milk in a fridge. Almond milk will keep up to a few days.

Serves: 4 cups

Ingredients:

- 4 cups filtered, preferably alkaline water
- 1 cup of raw almonds
- half teaspoon Himalayan salt or sea salt
- stevia to swecten if needed

Instructions:

1. First, soak almonds in water with half teaspoon salt (sea salt or Himalayan salt) for about 12 hours.
2. Place in a high-speed blender until the mixture is smooth.
3. Strain using cheesecloth.
4. Place in a blender again, adding some stevia to sweeten if needed.
5. Stir well and place in a fridge.
6. Serve with a splash of lemon or lime juice or some fresh cinnamon. So yummy, healthy and nutritious!

Raw Coconut Milk

I realize that some people may be allergic to nuts, or for whatever reason, don't like them. I want to invite you to try some homemade raw coconut milk instead. Just like almond milk, you can use it in cooking, baking, smoothies, and other natural drinks. You can experiment with cocoa, vanilla, dried fruits, and strawberries to give it some flavor.

Serves: 4
Ingredients:
- 4 cups of warm water
- 2 cups shredded coconut

Instructions:
1. I recommend you make this recipe in 2 batches.
2. First, take 1 cup of coconut and 2 cups of water and place in a blender. Keep blending for a few minutes until smooth.
3. Strain using a colander and set aside. Keep the strained coconut as well. You can use it for desserts or add it back to your milk.
4. Now, blend the second batch. Place another 2 cups of water and 1 cup of shredded coconut in the blender.
5. Blend well.

6. Mix the two batches and, if needed, add some of the blended coconut for more thickness.

7. Sweeten with stevia if needed.

8. Enjoy!

BONUS RECIPES: Fruit Infused Spa Water Recipes for Wellness, Detoxification and Weight Loss

Citrus and Basil Romance

Serves: 4

Ingredients:

- 1 liter of water (4 cups)
- 1 orange, sliced
- 1 lime, sliced
- 1 grapefruit, sliced
- ¼ cup of fresh basil leaves

Instructions:

1. In a jar, mix water with fruits and basil.
2. Stir gently and press.
3. Cover and place in a fridge for 1 hour (citrus fruits are fast to infuse so it can be less than 1 h, see what works for you).
4. Serve with some nice ice cubes.
5. Enjoy!

Beets Spa Water

Serves: 4

Ingredients:

- 2 beets, sliced
- Half cup of cherry tomatoes, sliced
- 2 kiwis, sliced
- Fresh mint leaves
- 1 liter of water (4 cups)

Instructions:

1. In a jar, mix water with tomatoes, beets, and kiwis.
2. Add some mint, stir, and press.
3. Cover and let cool down for a few hours.
4. Serve with some fresh lime or lemon juice and a few ice cubes of your choice. Enjoy!

Red Grape VIP Spa Water

If you have some friends over and you want to enjoy a few glasses of wine, it's also good to have some healthy soft drinks at hand.

This one is one of my favorites, and all my friends love it!

Serves: 4

Ingredients:

- 1 liter of water
- 1 cup of red grapes
- 1 teaspoon maple syrup
- 2 lemons, sliced
- A few basil leaves

Instructions:

1. In a jar, mix water with grapes and lemons.
2. Add maple syrup and basil.
3. Stir and press.
4. Cover and cool down in a fridge for a few hours.
5. Serve with a few ice cubes.
6. Enjoy!

Creating a Healthy Lifestyle You Love

Don't wait. Take <u>meaningful and purposeful</u> action today. You already know that you need to add more alkaline foods into your diet. Here are a few simple steps that you can implement to feel more energized while improving your wellbeing:

- Try to have at least 1 alkaline smoothie a day. Juicing vegetables is also great. With one smoothie and one juice a day you will succeed sooner than you think (check out my other books such as: *Alkaline Drinks* and *Alkaline Juicing* for juicing recipes)

- Try to have at least 1 big salad a day. You can also start adding more greens to your other meals. Again, this does not mean that you should live on greens and green salads alone. But you should get in a habit of serving massive portions of leafy green veggies with your meals. You can try some recipes from my book *Alkaline Salads*

- Drink plenty of filtered alkaline water. You can purchase a water pitcher, which will help you save money in the long run. Most bottled water brands have an acidifying effect on our body. Switching to alkaline water will be the best health investment you have ever made. A good water pitcher can be ordered for less than

$100. Then, all you need to do is periodically change the filters.

- Going alkaline does not mean you have to go 100% plant-based (of course you can, and I will support your decision). However, it does encourage you to reduce animal products. There are many other plant-based options that are easy to make, nutritious and delicious. Also, looking for more plant-based options (even if you are not vegan), stimulates creativity.

- Reduce caffeine. As soon as you start adding more alkaline foods into your diet, your energy levels will skyrocket.

- Ask yourself everyday how you can add more veggies, especially raw veggies, into your diet.

- Move your body. If you are not a gym person, start going for long, revitalizing walks (one of my favorite activities!). Ask a friend to accompany you, if you feel like this will help you get and stay motivated. You can also combine your walks with a social life; just call a friend or create your health group via meetup.com.

- Relax, practice mindfulness, and live in the NOW. Most of our "Western society" problems are nothing compared to what people in other countries experience. We have everything. We should be grateful, not complaining. Mind that the alkaline diet lifestyle is not only about what you eat and drink. It's also about how you live and what you think.

- Spend more time embracing your hobbies and things you enjoy doing. You deserve more self-care!

Don't forget to sign up for our email newsletter to get instant access to your bonuses:

ww.holisticwellnessproject.com/alkaline

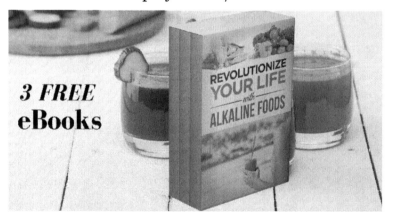

More Books Written by Marta

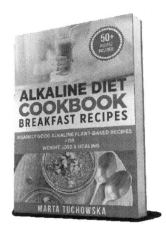
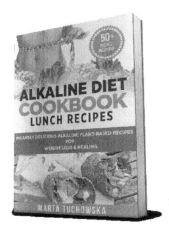

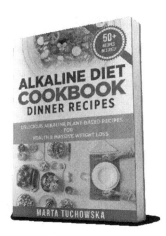
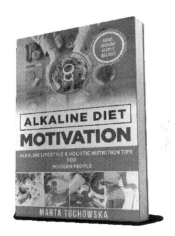

Available on Amazon:

www.amazon.com/author/mtuchowska

You will find more at:

www.holisticwellnessproject.com/books

Thanks again for your time and interest in my work.

It was a pleasure to "talk" to you,

I hope we "meet" again soon!

In the meantime, let's connect:

www.instagram.com/Marta_Wellness

www.facebook.com/HolisticWellnessProject

www.HolisticWellnessProject.com

I wish you wellness, health, and success in whatever it is that you want to accomplish.

Marta Tuchowska

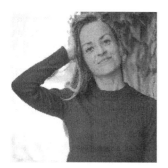

PS. Before you go, could you please do something for me? If you received any value from this book, could you please post a short review and let others know about your experience? It will help more readers take better care of their wellbeing and enjoy the energizing benefits of alkaline smoothies. It will only take a few seconds. It's you I am writing for and I would love to hear from you in the review section of this book!

Made in the USA
Middletown, DE
14 September 2019